Thai Cuisine for Beginners

Quick and Easy Recipes to Discover Thai Cooking and
Boost Your Taste

Tim Singhapat

Table of contents

FRIED WON TONS

Ingredients:

- ½ cup chopped white mushrooms
  ½ pound ground pork
- 1 clove garlic, minced
- 1 tablespoon soy sauce
- 2 tablespoons minced cilantro
- 25 won ton skins
- Pinch white pepper
- Vegetable oil for frying

Directions:

1. In a moderate-sized-sized mixing container, meticulously mix the garlic, cilantro, soy sauce, mushrooms, white pepper, and ground pork.
2. To make the won tons, place roughly ½ teaspoon of the filling in the center of a won ton skin. Fold the won ton from corner to corner, making a triangle. Push the edges together to secure closed. Repeat with the rest of the skins and filling.
3. Put in approximately two to three inches of vegetable oil to a deep fryer or wok. Heat the oil on medium until it reaches about 350 degrees. Cautiously add the won tons, 2 or 3 at a time. Fry until they become golden brown, turning them continuously. Move the cooked won tons to drain using paper towels as they are done.
4. Serve the won tons with either sweet-and-sour sauce or the sauce of your choice.

Yield: Approximately 25 won tons

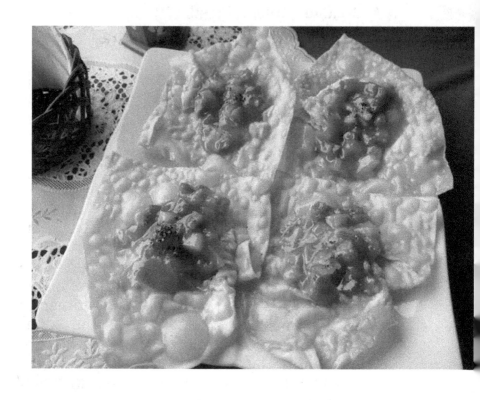

MEE KROB

Ingredients:

- ½ cup dried shrimp
- ½ pound thin rice stick noodles, broken into handfuls 1 cup bean sprouts
- 1 tablespoon Tamarind Concentrate (Page 20)
  10 small lime wedges
- 2 eggs, beaten
- 2–3 drops red food coloring
- 5 tablespoons sugar
- 1 cup honey
- 1 cup rice or white vinegar
- Vegetable oil for deep-frying

Directions:

1. Mix the honey, vinegar, sugar, food coloring, and tamarind in a moderate-sized deep cooking pan. Bring the mixture to its boiling point on moderate heat, stirring once in a while. Decrease the heat and simmer for two to three minutes or until the mixture starts to thicken; turn off the heat and save for later.
2. Bring about 3 inches of vegetable oil to 360 degrees in a deep fryer or frying pan. Drop a single layer of the rice stick noodles into the hot oil, ensuring to leave enough room for them to cook uniformly. Turn the noodles using a slotted spoon the moment they start to puff up. Once the noodles are golden,

remove them to paper towels to drain. Repeat until all of the noodles are cooked.

3. Put in the dried shrimp to the oil and cook for 45 seconds or so. Remove to paper towels.

4. Pour out all but a thin coat of the oil from the frying pan. Put in the beaten eggs and stir-fry them swiftly, shirring them into lengthy strips. Once they are cooked, remove them to paper towels.

5. Bring the sauce back to its boiling point. Mix in the shrimp and continue to boil for a couple of minutes.

6. Put about of the noodles on a serving platter and spoon about of the sauce over the top; lightly toss to coat the noodles uniformly being cautious not to crush the noodles. Repeat until all of the noodles are coated in sauce.

7. To serve, mound the noodles, put the egg strips over them, and top with the bean sprouts. Pass the lime wedges.

Yield: Servings 4–6

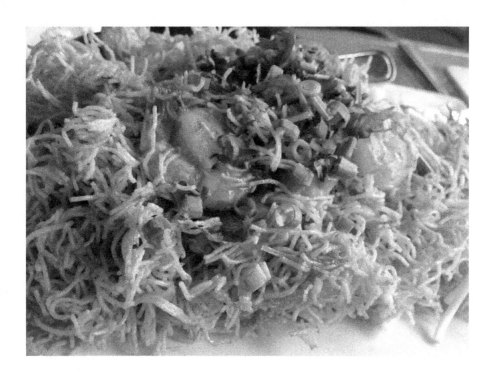

OMELET "EGG ROLLS"

Ingredients:

For the filling:

- ½ pound ground pork or chicken
- ½ teaspoon sugar
- 1 cup shredded Chinese cabbage
- 1 tablespoon fish sauce
- 1 tablespoon minced cilantro
- 1 teaspoon vegetable oil
- 2 green onions, trimmed and thinly cut

For the omelets:

- 1 tablespoon soy or fish sauce
- 1 teaspoon vegetable oil
- 6 tablespoons water
- 8 eggs
- Bibb lettuce
- Decorate of your choice
- Soy sauce, fish sauce, and/or hot sauce

Directions:

1. To make the filling: In a moderate-sized-sized frying pan, warm the vegetable oil on moderate heat. Put in the ground meat and sauté until it is no longer pink. Put in the green onions and cabbage and cook until tender. Put in the sugar, fish sauce, and cilantro; cook for 1 more minute. Set the filling aside, keeping it warm.
2. To make the omelets: Mix the eggs, water, and soy sauce in a moderate-sized

container. Put an omelet pan on moderate heat for a minute. Put in roughly ¼ teaspoon of vegetable oil, swirling it to coat the pan uniformly. Pour roughly ¼ of the egg mixture into the pan, then allow it to rest for roughly half a minute. When the bottom is firm, flip the omelet and cook until done. Transfer to a plate and cover using foil to keep warm. Repeat to make 3 more omelets.

3. To fill the "Egg Rolls," place 1 omelet in the middle of a plate. Put ¼ of the filling slightly off-center and then roll up. Trim the ends and chop the rolls into bite-sized pieces.

4. To serve, use Bibb lettuce leaves to pick up the rolls. Immerse in additional soy sauce, fish sauce, hot sauce, or other favorite dipping sauce, and put in the decorate of your choice.

Yield: 16–20 pieces

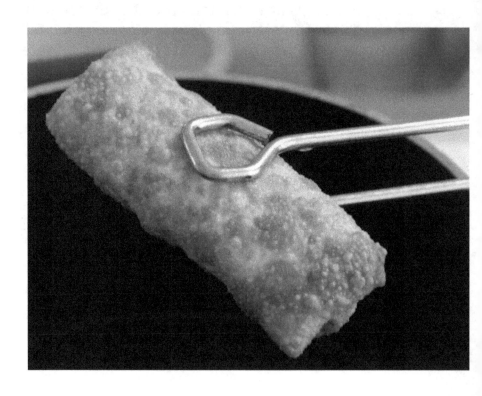

PORK TOAST TRIANGLES

Ingredients:

- ¼ pound of big shrimp, peeled and deveined 1
- egg
- 1 pound ground pork (the leaner the better)
- 1 tablespoon chopped cilantro
- 1 tablespoon dried shrimp
- 1 tablespoon fish sauce
- 2 cloves garlic, peeled
  6 slices day-old bread, crusts trimmed off
- Vegetable oil for
- frying

Directions:

1. Fill a moderate-sized deep cooking pan with water and bring it to its boiling point. Reduce the heat, put in the shrimp, and simmer until the shrimp are opaque. Drain the shrimp and let cool completely. Coarsely cut and save for later.
2. Put the dried shrimp, cilantro, and the garlic in a food processor and pulse until a smooth paste is formed. Put in the reserved shrimp and ground pork; process once more. Put in the egg and fish sauce and process one more time.
3. Spread the mixture uniformly over each slice of bread. Chop the bread into 4 equal

slices, either from corner to corner forming triangles or from top to bottom forming squares.

4. Put in roughly ½ inch of vegetable oil to a big frying pan. Bring the oil to roughly 375 degrees on moderate to high heat. Put 4 to 5 toasts in the oil, filling side down. Ensure that the toasts are not crowded in the oil or they will not brown uniformly. After the filling side is well browned, use a slotted spoon or metal strainer to flip the toasts. Watch the toasts cautiously, as the bottoms will brown swiftly. Take away the toasts to a stack of paper towels to drain. Cautiously pat the tops of the toasts using paper towels to remove any oil.

5. Serve the toasts with sweet-and-sour or plum sauce.

Yield: 24 pieces

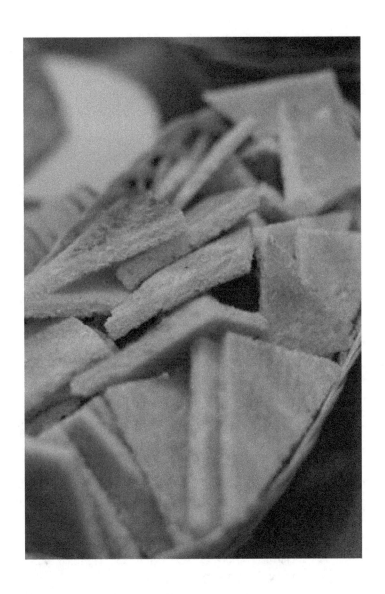

PORK, CARROT, AND CELERY SPRING ROLLS

Ingredients:

- ¼ cup fish sauce
- ¼ teaspoon white pepper
- 1 cup bean sprouts
- 1 cup minced or ground pork
- 1 teaspoon minced garlic
- 2 cups chopped celery
- 2 cups grated carrots
- 2 egg yolks, beaten
- 2 tablespoons sugar
- 2 tablespoons vegetable oil
- 20 spring roll wrappers
- Vegetable oil for deep frying

Directions:

1. In a big frying pan, heat the 2 tablespoons of vegetable oil over moderatehigh heat. Put in the garlic and pork, and sauté until the pork is thoroughly cooked.
2. Put in the carrots, celery, fish sauce, sugar, and white pepper. Increase heat to high and cook for a minute.
3. Drain any liquid from the pan and allow the mixture to cool completely, then mix in the bean sprouts.
4. On a clean, dry work surface, put the egg roll wrapper with an end pointing toward you, making a diamond. Put roughly 2 tablespoons of the filling on the lower portion of the wrapper. Fold up the corner nearest

you and roll once, then fold in the sides. Brush the rest of the point with the egg yolk and finish rolling to secure. Repeat with the rest of the wrappers and filling.
5. Heat 2 to 3 inches of oil to 350 degrees. Deep-fry the spring rolls until a golden-brown colour is achieved; remove instantly to drain using paper towels.
6. Serve with sweet-and-sour sauce.

Yield: 20 rolls

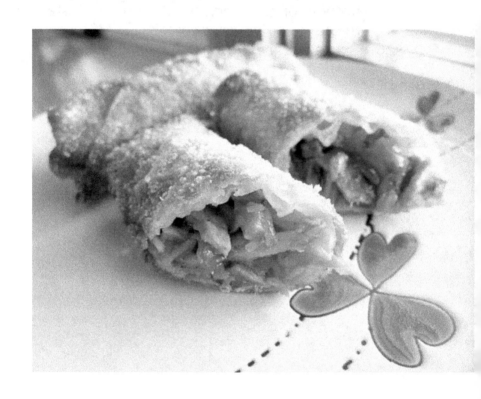

RICE PAPER ROLLS

Ingredients:

- 1 cup thin rice noodles
- 4 (8" × 10") sheets of rice paper
- 1 cup grated carrot
- 2 scallions, thinly cut
- 1 small cucumber, shredded 20 mint leaves
- 1 small bunch cilantro
  8–10 medium to big cooked shrimp, cut in
- half

Directions: Soak the rice noodles in super hot water until they are soft, usually ten to twenty minutes; drain. You can leave the noodles whole, or cut them into two-inch pieces if you prefer.

1. Put a sanitized kitchen towel on a work surface with a container of hot water nearby. Place a sheet of the rice paper in the hot water for roughly twenty seconds, just until soft; lay it out flat on the towel.
2. In the center of the rice paper, place 2 to 3 pieces of shrimp and ¼ of the noodles, carrots, scallions, and cucumbers. Top with mint and cilantro.
3. Swiftly roll up the rice paper, keeping it quite tight; then roll up the whole thing using plastic wrap, ensuring to keep it tight. Place in your fridge until ready to serve.
4. To serve, trim the ends off the rolls. Chop the remaining roll into pieces and remove the plastic wrap. Serve with a dipping sauce of your choice.

Yield: Servings 2–4

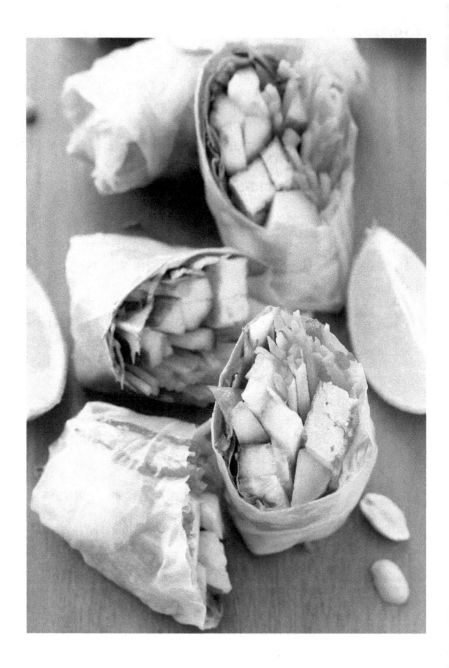

SALT-CURED EGGS

Ingredients:

- 1 dozen eggs
- 1½ cups salt
- 6 cups water

Directions:

1. Mix the water and the salt in a big deep cooking pan and bring to its boiling point using high heat. Turn off the heat and let cool completely.
2. Cautiously place the eggs in a container. Pour the salt water over the eggs and seal the container firmly. Put the container in your fridge and let the eggs cure for minimum 1 month.
3. To serve, hard-boil the eggs, let cool completely, then peel, slice, and enjoy.

Yield: 1 dozen eggs

SHRIMP TOAST

Ingredients:

- ¼ pound ground pork
- ¼ teaspoon salt
- ½ pound shrimp, cleaned, deveined, and crudely chopped 1 egg, beaten
- 1 tablespoon chopped cilantro
- 2 cloves garlic, minced
- 2 tablespoons sesame seeds
- 2 teaspoons soy sauce
- 2 teaspoons vegetable oil, divided
- 32 slices cucumber
- 8 slices of white bread, left to sit out overnight, crusts removed teaspoon
- cayenne

Directions:

1. In a small container, mix the shrimp and pork; set aside.
2. In another small container, mix the cilantro, garlic, cayenne, and salt. Pour the spice mixture over the shrimp and pork, and combine.
3. Mix in the beaten egg and soy sauce; mix thoroughly. Split the mixture into 8 parts.
4. Smoothly spread a slim layer of the mixture on each slice of bread and drizzle with sesame seeds.
5. Heat ¼ teaspoon vegetable oil in nonstick frying pan. When it is super hot, place 1 piece of bread, meat side down, in the oil. Cook until golden in color, then remove to a paper towel, blotting any surplus oil. Repeat for all of the bread sides.

6. Cut each slice of bread into four equivalent portions and top each quarter with a cucumber slice.

Yield: 32 pieces

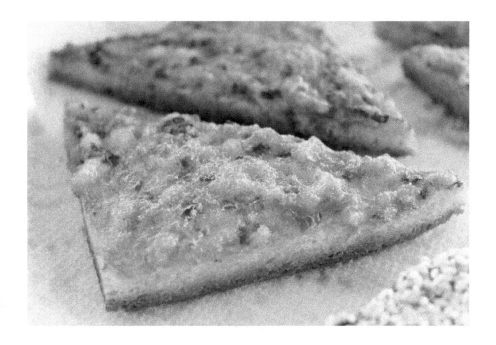

SKEWERED THAI PORK

Ingredients:

- 1 pound pork, thinly cut into lengthy strips
- 1 tablespoon coconut milk
- 1 tablespoon fish sauce
- 1 teaspoon salt
- 2 tablespoons sugar
- 20–30 bamboo skewers, soaked in water for an hour 3 cloves
- garlic, minced

Directions:

1. In a moderate-sized-sized container, mix the sugar, salt, garlic, fish sauce, and coconut milk.
2. Toss the pork strips in the mixture to coat completely. Cover the container and marinate for minimum 30 minutes, but if possible overnight in your fridge.
3. Thread the pork strips onto the bamboo skewers.
4. Grill the skewers for approximately 3 to five minutes per side.
5. Serve with your favorite sauce or as is.

Yield: Servings 2–3

SON-IN-LAW EGGS

Ingredients:

- ¼ cup chopped cilantro
- ¼ cup vegetable oil
- 10 hard-boiled eggs, cooled and peeled
- 2 shallots, thinly cut
- 3 tablespoons fish sauce
- 1 cup light brown sugar
- 1 cup Tamarind Concentrate (Page 20)
- Dried hot chili flakes to taste

Directions:

1. Heat the vegetable oil in a frying pan on moderate heat. Put the whole eggs in the frying pan and fry until a golden-brown colour is achieved. Take away the eggs to paper towels and save for later. (If your frying pan can't hold all of the eggs easily, do this in batches.)
2. Put in the shallots to the frying pan and sauté until just starting to brown. Take away the shallots from the oil using a slotted spoon and save for later.
3. Place the brown sugar, fish sauce, and tamarind in the frying pan. Stir to blend and bring to a simmer. Cook the mixture, stirring continuously, until the sauce thickens, approximately five minutes; turn off the heat.
4. Chop the eggs in half vertically and put them face-up on a rimmed serving dish. Spread the shallots over the eggs and then

sprinkle the eggs with the sauce. Decorate using cilantro and chili pepper flakes.

Yield: 20

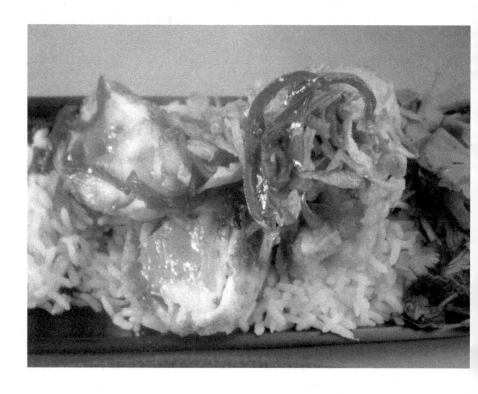

SPICY COCONUT BUNDLES

Ingredients:

- ½ cup chopped lime segments
- ½ cup chopped peanuts
- ½ cup diced red onion
- ½ cup dried shrimp
- 1 cup shredded fresh coconut
- 1–2 jalapeños, seeded and cut
  20–25 moderate-sized spinach leaves,
- washed and patted dry
- 1 cup brown sugar
- 1 cup shrimp paste

Directions:

1. Put the coconut in a moderate-sized sauté pan and cook on moderate heat until browned, approximately twenty minutes; allow to cool.
2. In a small deep cooking pan, melt the brown sugar on moderate heat, stirring continuously. Stir in the shrimp paste until well blended. Set the sauce aside.
3. Put the coconut, onion, lime pieces, peanuts, dried shrimp, and jalapeños in a moderate-sized serving container; lightly toss to blend.
4. To serve, place four to 5 spinach leaves (depending on the size of the leaves) on each serving plate. Top each leaf with roughly 1 tablespoon of the coconut mixture and sprinkle a small amount of sauce over the coconut.

5. To eat, roll up the spinach leaf around the coconut mixture and pop the whole bundle in your mouth. Pass additional sauce separately.

Yield: Servings 4

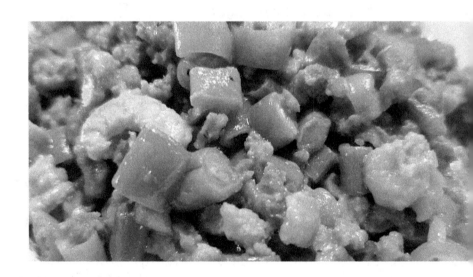

SPICY GROUND PORK IN BASIL LEAVES

Ingredients:

- ¼ tablespoon (or to taste) ground dried chili pepper
- ½ pound ground pork
- 1 shallot, thinly cut
- 1 tablespoon toasted rice powder (available in Asian specialty stores)
- 3 tablespoons fish sauce
- 5 sprigs cilantro, chopped
- Juice of 1–2 limes
- Lettuce and/or big basil leaves

Directions:

1. Squeeze the juice of half of a lime over the ground pork and let marinate for a few minutes.
2. Heat a big frying pan on high. Put in a couple of tablespoons of water and then instantly put in the pork; stir-fry until the pork is thoroughly cooked. (It is okay if the pork sticks at first — it will ultimately loosen.)
3. Pour off any fat that has collected in the pan and then put the pork in a big mixing container. Put in the remaining lime juice (to taste), fish sauce, shallot, ground chili pepper, cilantro, and toasted rice; stir until blended meticulously.
4. To serve, put the mixture in a serving container and let guests use the lettuce and basil leaves to scoop out the mixture.

Yield: Servings 4

SPICY SCALLOPS

Ingredients:

- 1 (½-inch) piece of ginger, peeled and minced
- 1 clove garlic, minced
- 1 jalapeño, seeded and minced
- 1 teaspoon vegetable oil
- 2 tablespoons soy sauce
- 2 tablespoons water
- 8 big scallops, cleaned
- teaspoon ground coriander

Directions:

1. In a pan big enough to hold all of the scallops, heat the oil on moderate heat. Put in the garlic, jalapeño, and ginger, and stir-fry for approximately one minute.
2. Put in the coriander, soy sauce, and water, stirring to blend; simmer for two to three minutes. Strain the liquid through a fine-mesh sieve. Allow the pan to cool slightly.
3. Put in the scallops to the pan and spoon the reserved liquid over the top of them. Return the pan to the stove, increasing the heat to moderate-high. Cover the pan and let the scallops steam for approximately two to three minutes, or until done to your preference. Serve instantly.

Yield: Servings 4

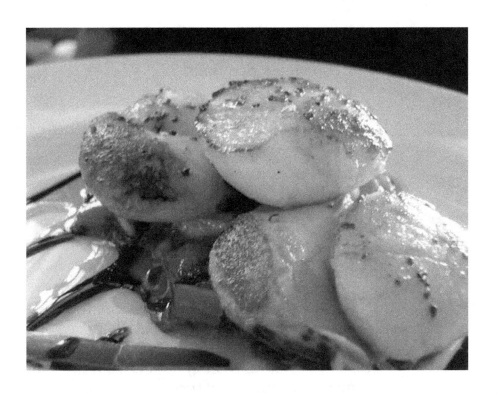

THAI FRIES

Ingredients:

- 1 14-ounce bag shredded sweetened coconut
- 1 cup rice flour
- 1 cup sticky rice flour
- 1 pound taro root
- 1 teaspoon black pepper
- 1 teaspoon salt
- 2 moderate-sized sweet potatoes
- 2 tablespoons sugar
- 3 tablespoons black sesame seeds
- 4 green plantains
- Water

Directions:

1. Peel the root vegetables and cut them into flat -inch-thick strips about 3 inches long and an inch wide.
2. Mix the flours in a big mixing container and mix in ½ cup of water. Continue putting in water ¼ cup at a time until a mixture resembling pancake batter is formed. Mix in rest of the ingredients.
3. Fill a moderate-sized deep cooking pan a third to a half full with vegetable oil. Heat the oil using high heat until super hot, but not smoking.
4. Put in some of the vegetables to the batter, coating them thoroughly. Using a slotted spoon or Asian strainer, put the vegetables in the hot oil. (Be careful here: The oil may

spatter.) Fry the vegetables, turning them once in a while, until a golden-brown colour is achieved. Move the fried vegetables to a stack of paper towels to drain, then serve instantly.

Yield: Servings 4–8

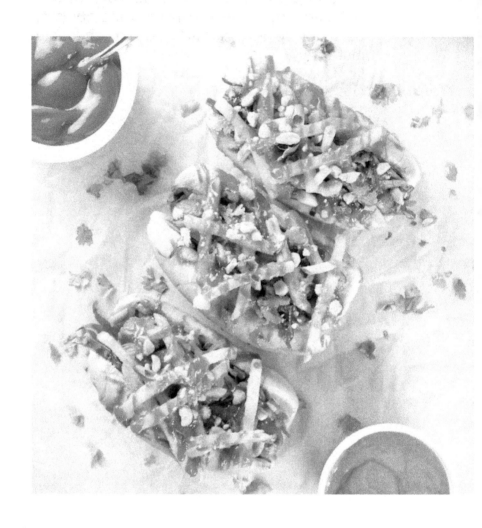

ASIAN CHICKEN NOODLE SOUP

Ingredients:

- ½ cup chopped onion
- 1 carrot, peeled and julienned
- 1 cup chopped cilantro
- 1 moderate-sized sweet red pepper, seeded and julienned
- 2 cups chicken broth
- 2 star anise
- 2 tablespoons chopped ginger
- 2 tablespoons fish sauce
- 2 tablespoons vegetable oil
- 2 whole boneless, skinless chicken breasts, cut into lengthy strips
- 3 cloves garlic, minced
- 3 ounces snow peas, trimmed
- 4 ounces, cellophane noodles, soaked in boiling water for five minutes and drained
- 5 cups water, divided
- Lemon or lime wedges
- Peanuts, crudely chopped

Directions:

1. In a big deep cooking pan, heat the oil on high. Put in the onion and sauté until translucent. Put in the ginger, garlic, and cilantro, and sauté for 1 more minute. Mix in the broth and 2 cups of the water. Put in the star anise. Bring to its boiling point, reduce heat, and cover; simmer for twenty minutes to half an hour.
2. In another deep cooking pan, bring the rest of the water to its boiling point. Put in the vegetables and blanch for a minute

or until soft-crisp. Drain and run very cold water over the vegetables to stop the cooking process; set aside.
3. Strain the broth into a clean soup pot and bring to its boiling point. Put in the chicken strips and reduce heat. Poach the chicken using low heat until opaque, roughly ten minutes. Put in the cellophane noodles and reserved vegetables, and carry on simmering for two more minutes. Season to taste with fish sauce.
4. To serve, ladle the soup into warm bowls. Drizzle with peanuts and decorate with lime wedge.

Yield: Servings 4 to 6

CHICKEN SOUP WITH LEMONGRASS

Ingredients:

- ¾ pound boneless, skinless chicken breast, trimmed and slice into bite-sized pieces
- 1 (14-ounce) can unsweetened coconut milk
- 1 (1-inch) piece ginger, cut into 6 pieces
- 1 clove garlic, minced
- 1 medium onion, minced
- 1 stalk lemongrass, trimmed, bruised, and slice into 2 to 3 pieces
- 1 tablespoon vegetable oil
- 2 cups wild or domestic mushrooms, cut into bite-sized pieces (if required)
- 2 tablespoons fish sauce
- 2 teaspoons prepared Red Curry Paste (Page 17) or curry powder
- 3 lime leaves (fresh or dried)
- 4 cups chicken broth
- Juice of 2 limes
- Salt and pepper to taste

Directions:

1. In a moderate-sized-sized deep cooking pan, mix the oil, onion, and garlic. Cook on moderate heat for a minute. Put in the lemongrass, curry paste, ginger, and lime leaves.
2. Cook while stirring, for about three minutes, then put in the broth. Bring to its boiling point, decrease the heat to

moderate, and carry on cooking for ten more minutes.
3. Put in the coconut milk, the chicken pieces, and the mushrooms. Continue to cook for five minutes or until the chicken is done.
4. Mix in the lime juice and fish sauce. Sprinkle salt and pepper to taste.
5. Take away the lemongrass, lime leaves, and ginger pieces before you serve.

Yield: Servings 4–6

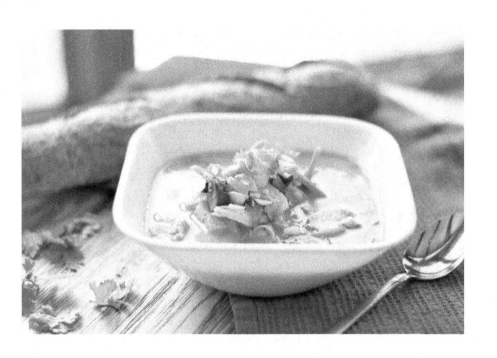

CHILLED MANGO SOUP

Ingredients:

- 1 cup plain yogurt
- 1 tablespoon dry sherry
- 1 teaspoon sugar (not necessary)
  1½ cups chilled chicken
  or vegetable broth 2
- big mangoes, peeled,
  pitted, and chopped
- Salt and white pepper
- to taste

Directions:

1. Put all of the ingredients in a blender or food processor and process until the desired smoothness is achieved. Adjust seasonings.
2. This soup may be served instantly or placed in the fridge until needed. If you do place in your fridge the soup, allow it to sit at room temperature for about ten minutes or so before you serve to take some of the chill off.

Yield: Servings 2–4

LEMONY CHICKEN SOUP

Ingredients:

- ½ cup lemon slices, including peel
- 1 cup straw mushrooms
- 1 tablespoon minced fresh ginger
- 1 whole boneless, skinless chicken breast, poached and shredded
- 1½ cups coconut milk
- 1½ teaspoons fresh hot chili pepper, seeded and chopped
- 1½ teaspoons sugar
- 2 cups chicken broth
- 2 green onions, thinly cut
- 3 tablespoons fish sauce
- 3 teaspoons lemongrass, peeled and chopped

Directions:

1. Mix the lemon slices, fish sauce, chili pepper, green onion, and sugar in a small glass container; set aside.
2. Mix the coconut milk, chicken broth, lemongrass, mushrooms, and ginger in a deep cooking pan. Bring to its boiling point, reduce heat, and simmer for twenty to twenty-five minutes. Put in the chicken and lemon mixture; heat through.
3. To serve, ladle into warmed bowls.

Yield: Servings 4–6

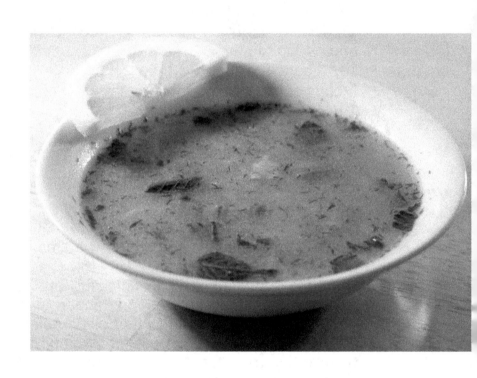

PUMPKIN SOUP

Ingredients:

For the broth:

- 1 clove of garlic, halved
- 1 moderate-sized leek, cut
- 1 red chili pepper, cut in half and seeded
- 1 small banana, cut
- 1 small pumpkin, peeled, seeded, and cut into little chunks
- 1 tablespoon finely chopped ginger
- 1 tablespoon Green Curry Paste
- 1½ stalks celery, cut
- 2 tablespoons butter
- 3 stalks lemongrass, peeled and thinly cut
- 3¼ cups vegetable broth
- 1 cup coconut milk
- 1 cup half-and-half
- Salt and pepper to taste

For the chicken and vegetables:

- ¾ cup cooked rice
- 1 small Japanese eggplant, cut into 4 pieces
- 1 tablespoon vegetable oil
- 1 whole boneless, skinless chicken breast, trimmed and slice into strips
- 2 kaffir lime leaves, cut into strips
- 2 red chili peppers, cut in half and seeded (not necessary)
- 2 tablespoons butter

- 2 teaspoons finely chopped ginger
- Green Curry Paste
- Thai basil

Yield: Servings 4

Directions:

1. In a big pot, melt the butter on moderate heat. Put in the pumpkin, leeks, celery, bananas, chili pepper, lemongrass, garlic, and ginger; sweat for five minutes.
2. In another sauté pan, heat the vegetable oil. Put in the eggplant and sauté until just warmed through.
3. Melt the butter in a heavy-bottomed sauté pan on moderate heat. Put in the chicken strips, ginger, lime leaves, and curry paste. Sauté until the chicken is cooked, but not browned. Put in the chicken mixture to the broth.
4. Put in the half-and-half, coconut milk, and curry paste; simmer for fifteen to twenty minutes.
5. Put in the vegetable broth and heat until warm.
6. Take away the chili pepper halves. Move the broth mixture to a blender or food processor and purée until the desired smoothness is achieved. Strain if you wish, and season to taste with salt and pepper. Pour the mixture into a clean pot and keep warm. To prepare the chicken and vegetables:
7. To serve, split the rice among 4 soup bowls. Ladle the broth over the rice. Top with a piece of eggplant, a chili pepper half (if you wish), and some basil.

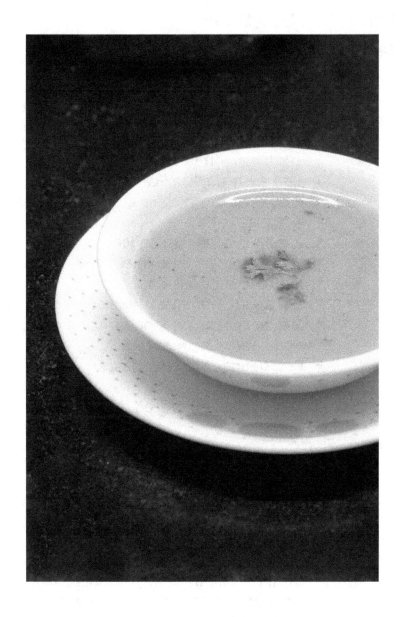

SPICY SEAFOOD SOUP

Ingredients:

- ¼ cup cut green onions
- 1 pound moderate-sized raw shrimp, peeled and deveined, shells reserved
- 1 quart water
- 1 tablespoon vegetable oil
- 10 (-inch-thick) slices fresh ginger
- 2 fresh serrano chilies, seeded and chopped
- 2 quarts fish or chicken stock
- 2 tablespoons fish sauce
- 2 tablespoons lime juice
- 24 fresh mussels, cleaned
- 3 stalks lemongrass, peeled and chopped
- 3 tablespoons chopped fresh cilantro
- 6–8 kaffir lime leaves
- Red pepper flakes to taste
- Salt
- Zest of 1 lime, grated

Directions:

1. Heat the vegetable oil in a big deep cooking pan. Put in the shrimp shells and sauté until they turn bright pink. Put in the stock, water, lemongrass, lime zest, lime leaves, ginger, and serrano chilies. Bring to its boiling point, reduce heat, and simmer for half an hour Strain the broth into a clean soup pot.
2. Bring the broth to its boiling point. Put in the mussels, cover, and cook until the shells open, approximately 2 minutes. Use a slotted

spoon to remove the mussels, discarding any that have not opened. Take away the top shell of each mussel and discard. Set aside the mussels on the half shell.

3. Put in the shrimp to the boiling broth and cook until they are opaque, approximately 2 minutes. Decrease the heat to low.
4. Put in the mussels to the pot. Mix in the lime juice, fish sauce, cilantro, red pepper flakes, and green onions. Simmer for one to two minutes. Season to taste with salt.
5. Serve instantly.

Yield: Servings 4–6

THAI-SPICED BEEF SOUP WITH RICE NOODLES

Ingredients:

- ¼ cup fish sauce
- ¾ cup leftover beef roast, chopped or shredded 1 (2–
- inch) cinnamon stick
- 1 stalk lemongrass, tough outer leaves removed, inner core crushed and minced
- 1 tablespoon prepared chiligarlic sauce
- 1 whole star anise, crushed
- 2 (¼–inch) pieces peeled gingerroot
- 2½ tablespoons lime juice
- 3–4 teaspoons (or to taste) salt
- 8 cups beef broth
- 8 ounces rice noodles, soaked in hot water for approximately ten minutes, strained and washed in cold water Freshly ground black
- pepper to taste

Directions:

1. In a moderate-sized-sized deep cooking pan, simmer the beef broth, star anise, cinnamon stick, and ginger using low heat for thirty to forty minutes.
2. Strain the stock and return to the deep cooking pan.
3. Put in the noodles, lemongrass, shredded beef, fish sauce, chili sauce, and garlic. Bring the soup to its boiling point on moderate heat. Decrease the heat and simmer for five minutes. Mix in the lime juice, salt, and pepper.

Yield: Servings 4–6

TOM KA KAI

Ingredients:

- 1 (1-inch) piece ginger, cut thinly
- 1 (2-inch) piece of lemongrass, bruised
- 1 boneless, skinless chicken breast, cut into bite-sized pieces
- 1 teaspoon cut kaffir lime leaves
- 2 cups chicken broth
- 2 tablespoons lime juice
- 2–4 Thai chilies (to taste), slightly crushed
- 4 tablespoons fish sauce
- 5 ounces coconut milk

Directions:

1. In a moderate-sized-sized soup pot, heat the broth on medium. Put in the lime leaves, lemongrass, ginger, fish sauce, and lime juice.
2. Bring the mixture to its boiling point, put in the chicken and coconut milk, and bring to its boiling point once more.
3. Reduce the heat, put in the chilies, and cover; allow to simmer until the chicken is thoroughly cooked, approximately 3 to five minutes.
4. Take away the chilies and the lemongrass stalk using a slotted spoon before you serve.

Yield: Servings 4–6

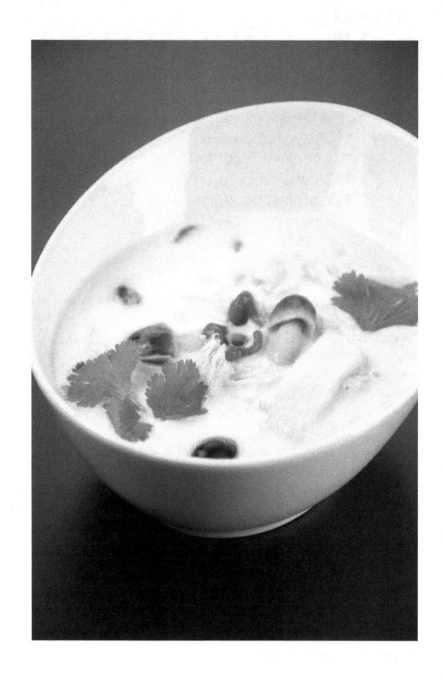

TOM YUM

Ingredients:

- 1 can straw mushrooms, drained
  2 stalks lemongrass, bruised and slice into 1-
- inch-long segments
- 2 tablespoons fish sauce
- 2 tablespoons minced fresh ginger
  20 moderate-sized shrimp, shelled
- but with tails left on 2–3 teaspoons
- cut kaffir lime leaves or lime zest
  2–3   Thai   chili
- peppers, seeded and
  minced   3   shallots,
- finely   chopped   3
- tablespoons lime juice
- 4–5 cups water

Directions:

1. Pour the water into a moderate-sized soup pot. Put in the shallots, lemongrass, fish sauce, and ginger. Bring to its boiling point, reduce heat, and simmer for about three minutes.
2. Put in the shrimp and mushrooms, and cook until the shrimp turn pink. Mix in the lime zest, lime juice, and chili peppers.
3. Cover and take out of the heat. Allow the soup to steep for five to ten minutes before you serve.

Yield: Servings 4–6

VEGETARIAN LEMONGRASS SOUP

Ingredients:

- ½ cup crudely shredded carrots
- ½ cup cut celery
- 1 can straw mushrooms, drained
- 1 cup snow peas, trimmed
- 1 red serrano chili, seeded and thinly cut
- 1 teaspoon (or to taste) crushed red peppers
- 4 tablespoons soy sauce
- 4–6 stalks lemongrass, bruised
- 8 cups low-sodium vegetable broth
- Juice of ½ lime or to taste

Directions:

1. Bring the broth to a simmer in a big deep cooking pan. Put in the crushed red peppers, lemongrass, soy sauce, and lime juice. Simmer for about ten minutes.
2. Put in the rest of the ingredients. Continue to simmer until the vegetables are just done, approximately two to three minutes. Take away the lemongrass stalks before you serve.

Yield: Servings 4–6

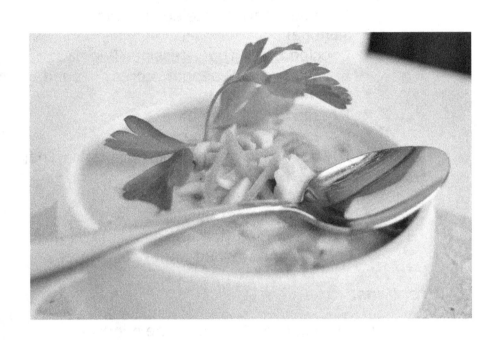

ASIAN NOODLE AND VEGETABLE SALAD

Ingredients:

- ¼ pound snow peas, trimmed and cut on the diagonal ½ cup
- toasted peanuts, chopped 1 cup
- bean sprouts
- 1 lime, cut into 6–8 wedges
- 1 medium carrot, peeled and thinly cut on the diagonal
- 1 recipe Spicy Thai Dressing (Page 33)
- 1 small red bell pepper, cored, seeded, and slice into fine strips
- 1 teaspoon sesame oil
- 1 teaspoon soy sauce
- 10 basil leaves, shredded (if possible Thai or lemon)
- 2 teaspoons vegetable oil
- 4 green onions, thinly cut
- 8 ounces dried rice noodles, cooked firm to the bite and washed under cold water

Directions:

1. In a big container, toss the noodles with the oils and the soy sauce.
2. Blanch the snow peas in boiling water for half a minute and then wash them under cold water.
3. Put in the snow peas, bell pepper, and the carrot to the noodles and toss.
4. Sprinkle the Spicy Thai Dressing (Page 33) over the noodle mixture to taste, put in the basil, half of the green onions, and

half of the bean sprouts, and toss thoroughly.
5. To serve, put the noodle salad on a chilled serving platter. Spread the rest of the green onions, remaining bean sprouts, and the peanuts over the top. Squeeze the juice of 2 lime wedges over the whole dish, and use the rest of the wedges as decorate. Serve instantly.

Yield: Servings 4–6

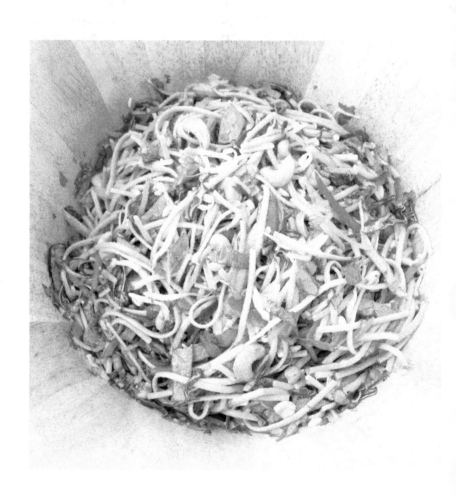

CRUNCHY COCONUT-FLAVORED SALAD

Ingredients:

- 1 cup julienned jicama
- 1 medium cucumber, peeled, seeded, and julienned
- 1 recipe Coconut Marinade (Page 12)
- 2–3 tablespoons chopped fresh basil

Directions:

1. Put the jicama, cucumber, and basil in a big container.
2. Pour the marinade over the vegetables and allow to rest in your fridge for minimum 2 hours before you serve.

Yield: Servings 2–3

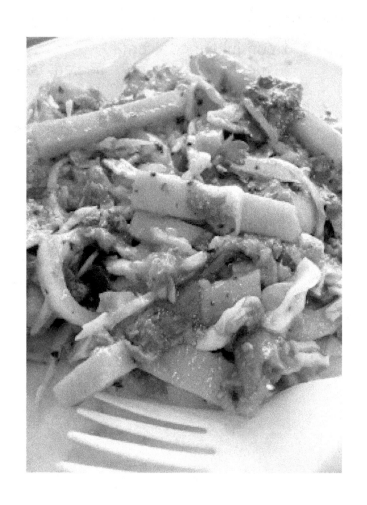

CUCUMBER SALAD WITH LEMONGRASS

Ingredients:

- ¼ cup minced mint
- ¼ cup minced parsley
- ½ cup shredded carrot
- ½ cup white vinegar
- 1 cup bean sprouts
- 1 cup cubed tart apple (such as Granny Smith)
- 1 garlic clove, very thoroughly minced
- 1 tablespoon fish sauce
- 1 tablespoon vegetable oil
- 1 Thai chili, very thoroughly minced
- 2 stalks lemongrass
- 3 cups thinly cut cucumber

Directions:

1. In a small deep cooking pan, mix the vinegar, chili, and garlic. Bring the mixture to its boiling point. Cover the pan, take it off the heat, and allow to cool.
2. Trim and finely cut 1 lemongrass stalk. Put it in a small deep cooking pan with ½ cup of water, cover, and bring to its boiling point. Turn off heat and allow to cool.
3. Trim the rest of the lemongrass stalk, peel off the tough outer layers, and finely mince the white portion of the soft stalk within. Reserve roughly 1 tablespoon.
4. Mix the cucumber, bean sprouts, apple, carrot, mint, and parsley in a big mixing container. In a small container mix the fish

sauce, oil, minced lemongrass, the vinegar mixture, and the lemongrass water.
5. Toss the vegetables with the lemongrass vinaigrette to taste.

Yield: Servings 6–8

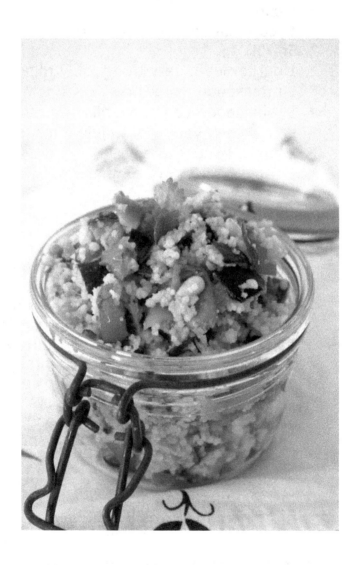

FIERY BEEF SALAD

Ingredients:

For the dressing:

- ¼ cup basil leaves
- ¼ cup lemon juice
- ¼ teaspoon black pepper
- 2 cloves garlic
- 2 tablespoons brown sugar
- 2 tablespoons chopped serrano chilies
- 2 tablespoons fish sauce

For the salad:

- ½ cup mint leaves
- 1 pound beef steak
- 1 small cucumber, finely cut
- 1 small red onion, finely cut
- 1 stalk lemongrass, outer leaves removed and discarded, inner stalk finely cut
- 1 tomato, finely cut
- Bibb or romaine lettuce leaves
- Salt and pepper to taste

Directions:

1. Mix all of the dressing ingredients in a blender and pulse until well blended; set aside.
2. Flavour the steak with salt and pepper. Over a hot fire, grill to moderate-rare (or to your preference). Move the steak to a platter, cover using foil, and allow to rest for five to ten minutes before carving.
3. Cut the beef across the grain into thin slices.

4. Put the beef slices, any juices from the platter, and the rest of the salad ingredients, apart from the lettuce, in a big mixing container. Put in the dressing and toss to coat.
5. To serve, place lettuce leaves on separate plates and mound the beef mixture on top of the lettuce.

Yield: Servings 2–4

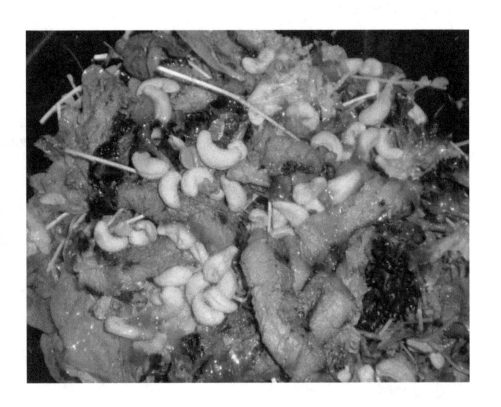

GRILLED CALAMARI SALAD

Ingredients:

For the dressing:
- 1 small onion, thinly cut
- 1 stalk lemongrass, inner core finely chopped
- 1 tablespoon fish sauce
- 1–5 red chili peppers, seeded and chopped
  3 kaffir lime leaves, chopped or 1 tablespoon
- lime zest
- 5 teaspoons lime juice
- 1 cup water

For the salad:

- 1 green onion, thinly cut
- 1 pound calamari, cleaned
- 6–8 sprigs cilantro, chopped
- Baby greens (not necessary)
- fifteen–20 mint leaves, chopped

Directions:

1. Mix all the dressing ingredients in a small container; set aside.
2. Prepare a grill or broiler. Put the calamari on a broiler pan or in a grill basket and cook using high heat until soft, approximately 3 minutes per side. Allow to cool to room temperature.
3. Put the grilled calamari in a mixing container. Mix the dressing and pour it over the calamari.

4. If serving instantly, put in the mint, cilantro, and green onions. If you don't like this method, allow the calamari to marinate for maximum 1 hour before you serve, and then put in the additional ingredients.
5. To serve: Use individual cups or bowls to help capture some of the wonderful dressing. If you don't like this method, mound the calamari mixture over a bed of baby greens and spoon additional dressing over the top.

Yield: Servings 2–4

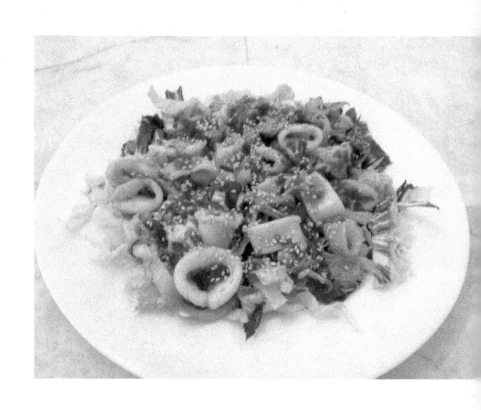

PAPAYA SALAD

Ingredients:

- ½ cup long beans (green beans), cut into 1-inch pieces ½-1
- teaspoon salt
- 1 medium papaya, peeled and julienned, or cut into little pieces
- 2 teaspoons fish sauce
- 2 tomatoes, thinly cut
- 3 jalapeño peppers, seeded and thinly cut
- 4 tablespoons <u>Tamarind Concentrate (Page 20)</u>
- 4-6 cloves of garlic, chopped crudely
- Sticky rice, cooked in accordance with package directions

Directions:

1. Put the papaya on a sheet pan and drizzle it with salt. Allow the papaya stand for half an hour Pour off any juice and then squeeze the fruit with your hands to extract as much fluid as you can. Put the pulp of the papaya in a big food processor.
2. Put in the chilies and pulse for a short period of time to blend. Put in the rest of the ingredients except the tomato and pulse again until combined.
3. Move the papaya mixture to a serving container and decorate with tomato slices. Serve with sticky rice.

Yield: Servings 4-6

SHRIMP AND NOODLE SALAD

Ingredients:

- ½–1 teaspoon dried red pepper flakes
- ¾ cup lime juice (roughly 4–5 limes)
- 1 clove garlic, minced
- 1 cup citrus fruit (oranges, grapefruit, tangerines, etc.) peeled, sectioned, and chopped
- 1 medium tomato, peeled, seeded, and chopped
- 1 stalk lemongrass, thoroughly minced (inner core only)
- 1 tablespoon brown sugar
- 1 tablespoon vegetable oil
- 2 tablespoons fish sauce
- 24 medium shrimp, peeled and deveined
- 3 green onions, cut
- 8 ounces rice noodles
- 1 cup chopped cilantro, plus extra for decoration
- 1 cup chopped mint leaves
- 1 cup chopped peanuts, plus extra for decoration Salt and
- ground pepper to taste

Directions:

1. Soak the rice noodles in hot water for ten to twenty minutes or until tender. While the noodles are soaking, bring a big pot of water to boil.
2. In the meantime, in a big container, combine the lemongrass, citrus, peanuts, tomato, scallions, mint, and cilantro.

3. In a small container, mix the red pepper flakes, garlic, sugar, lime juice, and fish sauce. (Adjust seasoning to your taste.)
4. Drain the noodles from their soaking liquid and put in them to the boiling water. When the water returns to its boiling point, drain them again and wash meticulously with cold water. Allow the noodles to drain well.
5. Put in the noodles and the dressing to the citrus mixture and toss to blend. Set aside.
6. Brush the shrimp with the vegetable oil and sprinkle with salt and pepper. Grill or sauté for roughly two minutes per side or until done to your preference.
7. To serve, mound the noodles in the middle of a serving platter. Put the grilled shrimp on top and decorate with peanuts and cilantro.

Yield: Servings 6

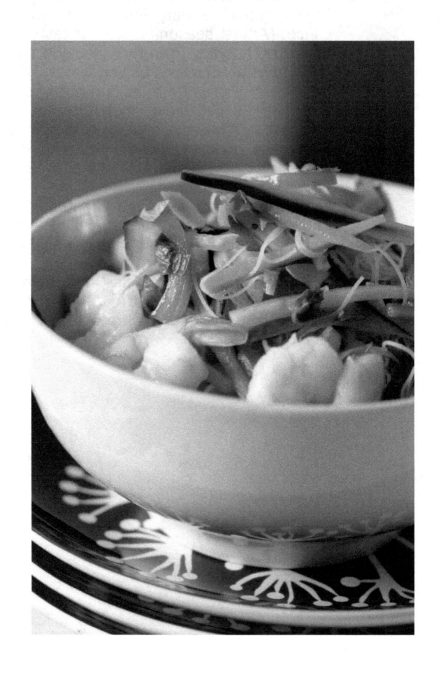

SPICY RICE SALAD

Ingredients:

For the dressing:

- ¼ cup hot chili oil
- ¼ cup lime juice
- ¼ cup sesame oil
- ½ cup fish sauce
- ½ cup rice vinegar

For the salad:

- 2 cups long-grained rice (if possible Jasmine)
- 2 carrots, peeled and diced
- 1 sweet red pepper, seeded and diced
- 1 serrano chili pepper, seeded and minced
- ¼–½ cup chopped mint ¼–½ cup
- chopped cilantro
- 1 pound cooked shrimp
- 1 cup chopped unsalted peanuts
- Lime wedges
- 4–6 green onions, trimmed and thinly cut

Directions:

1. Whisk together all of the dressing ingredients; set aside.
2. Cook the rice in accordance with the package directions. Fluff the rice, then move It to a blg mlxlng conLainer. Allow Lhe rice Lo cool slightly.
4. Pour roughly of the dressing over the rice and fluff to coat. Continue to fluff the rice

every so frequently until it is completely cooled.Put in the green onions, carrots, red pepper, serrano chili pepper, mint, cilantro, and shrimp to the rice. Toss with the rest of the dressing to taste.

5. To serve, place on separate plates and decorate with peanuts and lime wedges.

Yield: Approximately 8 cups

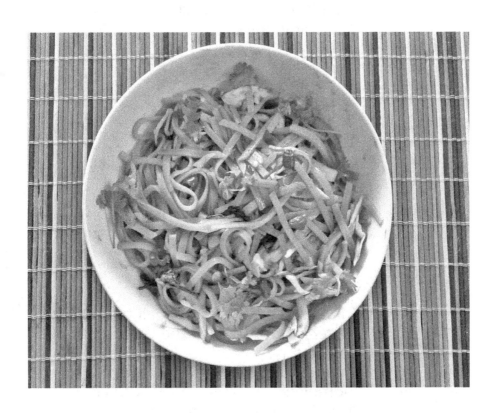

SPICY SHRIMP SALAD

Ingredients:

For the dressing:

- 2 tablespoons prepared chili sauce
- 3 tablespoons sugar
- 4 tablespoons fish sauce
- 1 cup lime juice

For the salad:

- ¼ cup chopped mint
- ¾ pound cooked shrimp
- 1 small red onion, thinly cut
- 2 cucumbers, peeled and thinly cut
- 2 green onions, trimmed and thinly cut Bibb
- lettuce leaves

Directions:

1. In a small container, mix all the dressing ingredients. Stir until the sugar dissolves completely.
2. In a big container, mix all of the salad ingredients apart from the lettuce. Pour the dressing over and toss to coat.
3. To serve, put the lettuce leaves on separate plates. Mound a portion of the shrimp salad on top of the leaves. Serve instantly.

Yield: Servings 2–4

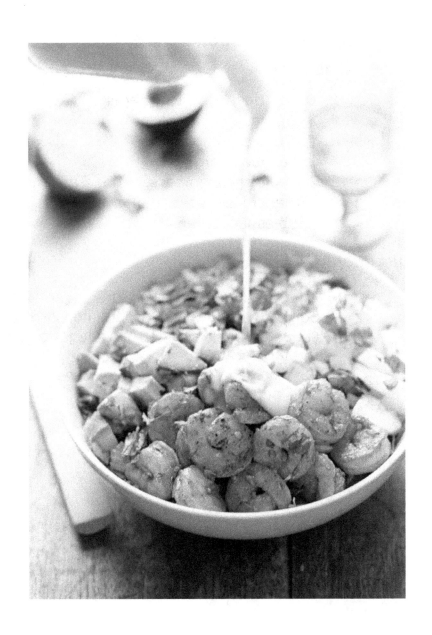

SWEET-AND-SOUR CUCUMBER SALAD

Ingredients:

- ½ cup rice or white vinegar
- 1 cup boiling water
- 1 small red onion, cut
- 1 teaspoon salt
- 2 medium cucumbers, seeded and cut
- 2 Thai chilies, seeded and minced
- 5 tablespoons sugar

Directions:

1. In a small container, mix the sugar, salt, and boiling water. Stir to meticulously dissolve sugar and salt. Put in the vinegar and allow the vinaigrette to cool completely.
2. Put the cucumbers, onion slices, and the chili peppers in a medium-sized container. Pour the dressing over the vegetables. Cover and let marinate in your fridge minimum until cold, if possible overnight.

Yield: Servings 2–4

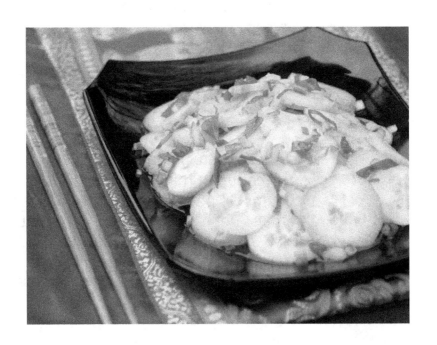

THAI DINNER SALAD

Ingredients:

For the dressing:

- ¾ teaspoon rice wine vinegar
- 1 clove garlic, minced
- 1 tablespoon lemon juice
- 1 tablespoon water
- 2 tablespoons fish sauce
- 2 teaspoons sugar
- Pinch of red pepper flakes

For the salad:

- ¼ cup chopped cilantro
- ¼ cup chopped mint leaves
- 1 cucumber, peeled, seeded, and diced
- 1 small head of romaine or Bibb lettuce, torn into bitesized pieces
- 2 small carrots, grated
- Chopped unsalted peanuts (not necessary)

Directions:

1. In a small container, mix together all of the salad dressing ingredients; set aside.
2. In a big container, toss together all of the salad ingredients. Put in dressing to taste and toss until thoroughly coated. Drizzle chopped peanuts over the top of each salad, if you wish.

Yield: Servings 2–4

THAILAND BAMBOO SHOOTS

Ingredients:

- 1 20-ounce can of bamboo shoots, shredded, liquid reserved
- 1 teaspoon fish sauce
- 1 teaspoon ground dried chili pepper
- 2 green onions, cut
- 2 tablespoons finely crushed peanuts, divided
- Juice of ½ lime
- Sticky rice, cooked in accordance with package directions

Directions:

1. Put the shredded bamboo shoots and roughly ¼ cup (half) of the reserved bamboo liquid in a moderate-sized deep cooking pan. Bring the contents of the pan to its boiling point, reduce heat, and allow to simmer until soft, approximately five minutes. Turn off the heat.
2. Mix in the lime juice, chili pepper, green onions, fish sauce, and 1 tablespoon of the peanuts.
3. Serve with sticky rice, sprinkled with the rest of the peanuts.

Yield: Servings 4

THAILAND SEAFOOD SALAD

Ingredients:

- ¼ cup fish sauce
- ½ pound salad shrimp
- ½ pound squid rings, poached in salted water for half a minute 1 (6-ounce) can chopped clams, drained 1 clove garlic,
- minced
-
- 1 green onion, trimmed and thinly cut
- 1 small onion, finely chopped
- 1 small serrano chili, seeded and finely chopped
- 1 stalk celery, cleaned and thinly cut
- 1 stalk lemongrass, outer leaves removed, inner core minced
- 2 medium cucumbers, peeled, halved, seeded, and super slimly cut
- 2 tablespoons chopped mint
- Bibb lettuce leaves
- Sugar to taste

Directions:

1. In a big mixing container, gently mix the squid, shrimp, clams, cucumber, and celery; set aside.
2. In a small mixing container, mix together the onion, lemongrass, serrano chili, mint, garlic, green onion, and fish sauce. Put in sugar to taste.
3. Pour the dressing over the seafood mixture, tossing to coat. Cover and

allow it to sit for minimum 30 minutes before you serve.
4. To serve, place lettuce leaves in the middle of four to 6 plates. Mound the seafood salad on top of the lettuce leaves.

Yield: Servings 4–6

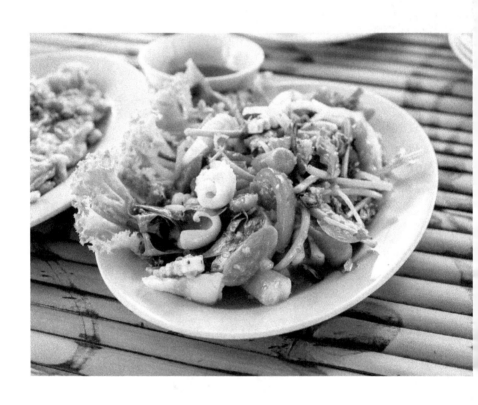

ZESTY MELON SALAD

Ingredients:

- ¼ cup honey
- ¼ teaspoon salt
- 1 serrano chili, seeded and minced (for a hotter salad, leave the seeds in)
- 2 cucumbers, peeled, halved, seeded, and cut
- 6 cups assorted melon cubes
- 6–8 tablespoons lime juice
- Zest of 1 lime

Directions:

1. In a big mixing container, mix the melon and the cucumber.
2. Combine the rest of the ingredients together in a small container. Pour over the fruit and toss thoroughly to coat.
3. Serve instantly, or if you prefer a zestier flavor, let the salad sit for maximum 2 hours to allow the chili flavor to develop.

Yield: Servings 4–6

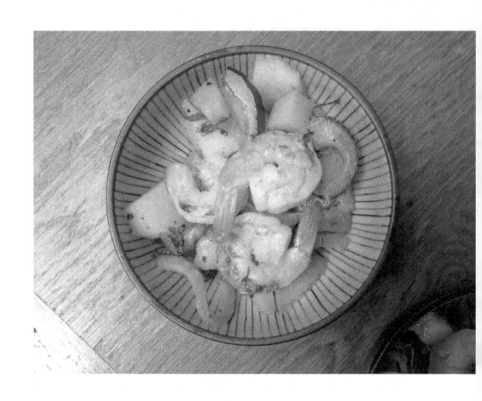

GREEN CURRY BEEF

Ingredients:

- ¼ cup (or to taste) Green Curry Paste
- ¼ cup brown sugar
- ¼ cup fish sauce
- 1 cup basil
- 1 pound eggplant (Japanese, Thai, or a combination), cut into ¼-inch slices
- 1½ pounds sirloin, cut into fine strips
- 2 cans coconut milk, thick cream separated from the milk
- 6 serrano chilies, stemmed, seeded, and cut in half along the length

Directions:

1. Put the thick cream from the coconut milk and the curry paste in a big soup pot and stir until blended. Put on moderate to high heat and bring to its boiling point. Decrease the heat and simmer for two to three minutes.
2. Put in the beef and the coconut milk, stirring to blend. Return the mixture to a simmer.
3. Put in the sugar and the fish sauce, stirring until the sugar dissolves, approximately 2 minutes.
4. Put in the eggplant and simmer for one to two minutes.
5. Put in the serrano chilies and cook one minute more.
6. Turn off the heat and mix in the basil.

Yield: Servings 4–6

CURRIED BEEF AND POTATO STEW

Ingredients:

- ¼ cup <u>Tamarind Concentrate</u> <u>(Page 20)</u>
- ½ cup brown sugar
- ½ cup unsalted roasted peanuts, chopped
- ½–¾ cup prepared <u>Massaman Curry Paste</u> <u>(Page 19)</u>
- 1 big onion, chopped
- 1 big russet potato, peeled and slice into bite-sized cubes
- 1 cup chopped fresh pineapple
- 1½ pounds beef stew meat, cut into bite-sized cubes 2 (14-ounce) cans coconut milk 2–3 tablespoons vegetable oil
- 7 tablespoons fish sauce
- Jasmine rice, cooked in accordance with package directions

Directions:

1. Heat the oil in a big soup pot on moderate to high heat. Once the oil is hot, brown the meat on all sides. Put in the onion and cook until translucent, approximately two to three minutes.
2. Put in enough water to just cover the meat and onions. Bring to its boiling point, reduce heat, cover, and simmer for thirty to 60 minutes.
3. Put in the potatoes and carry on simmering for fifteen more minutes. (The potatoes will not be fairly thoroughly cooked now.)

4. Strain the solids from the broth, saving for later both.
5. In another soup pot, mix the coconut milk with the curry paste until well mixed. Bring the contents to a simmer on moderate to high heat and cook for two to three minutes.
6. Put in the reserved meat and potato mixture, the sugar, fish sauce, and tamarind, stirring until the sugar dissolves. Put in some of the reserved broth to thin the sauce to desired consistency.
7. Mix in the pineapple and carry on simmering until the potatoes are thoroughly cooked.
8. To serve, place some Jasmine rice in the center of individual serving plates and spoon the stew over the top. Decorate using the chopped peanuts.

Yield: Servings 4

RED BEEF CURRY

Ingredients:

- ¼ cup chopped basil
- ½ cup plus 2 tablespoons coconut milk
- 1 green or red sweet pepper, seeded and cubed
- 1 pound lean beef, cut into fine strips
- 1 tablespoon vegetable oil
- 1–3 tablespoons (to taste) fish sauce
- 2 tablespoons (roughly) ground peanuts
- 2 tablespoons Red Curry Paste (Page 17)
- Rice, cooked in accordance with package directions Sugar
- to taste

Directions:

1. Heat the oil in a big sauté pan using low heat. Put in the curry paste and cook, stirring continuously, until aromatic, approximately one minute.
2. Mix in the ½ cup of coconut milk and bring the mixture to a simmer. Put in the beef strips and poach for five minutes.
3. Put in the peanuts and continue to poach for another five minutes.
4. Put in the fish sauce and sugar to taste; carry on cooking until the mixture is almost dry, then put in the sweet pepper and basil and cook for 5 more minutes.
5. Serve with rice.

Yield: Servings 4

HOT AND SOUR BEEF

Ingredients:

- 1 green onion, trimmed and thinly cut
- 1 tablespoon dark, sweet soy sauce
- 1 tablespoon fish sauce
- 1 tablespoon lime juice
- 1 teaspoon chopped cilantro
- 1 teaspoon dried chili powder
- 1 teaspoon honey
- 1½ pound sirloin steak
- 3 tablespoons chopped onion
- Salt and pepper to taste

Directions:

1. Make the sauce by meticulously combining the first 8 ingredients; set aside.
2. Flavour the steak with salt and pepper, then grill or broil it to your preferred doneness. Take away the steak from the grill, cover using foil, and allow to rest for five to ten minutes.
3. Thinly slice the steak, cutting across the grain.
4. Position the pieces on a serving platter or on 1 or 2 dinner plates. Ladle the sauce over the top. Serve with rice and a side vegetable.

Yield: Servings 1–2

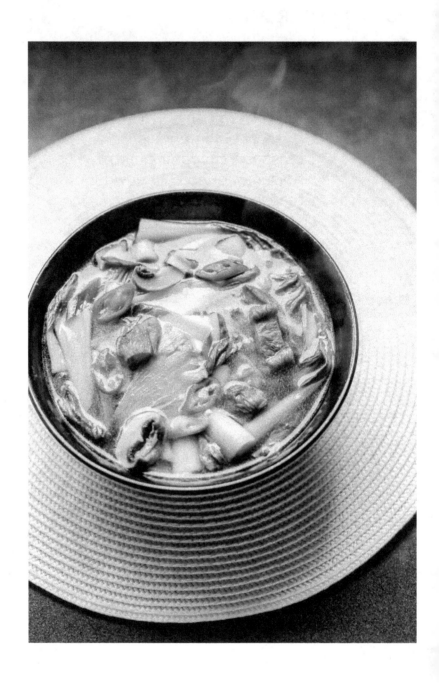

GRILLED GINGER BEEF
Ingredients:

- 1 (2-inch) piece of ginger, minced
- 1 (3-inch) piece ginger, cut in half
- 1 cinnamon stick
- 1 onion, cut in half
- 1 pound green vegetables
- 1 small package of rice noodles
- 2 dried red chili peppers
- 2 stalks lemongrass
- 2 tablespoons (or to taste) soy sauce
- 5 cloves garlic
- 6 (6-ounce) strip steaks
- 6 scallions, minced
- 8 cups low-salt beef broth
- Salt and pepper to taste

Directions:

1. Put the beef broth, lemongrass, and garlic in a big pot; bring to its boiling point.
2. Meanwhile, put the ginger and onion halves, cut-side down, in a dry frying pan using high heat and cook until black. Put in the onion and ginger to the broth mixture.
3. Put the cinnamon and dried chili peppers in the dry frying pan and toast on moderate heat for a minute; put in to the broth mixture.
4. Lower the heat and simmer the broth for a couple of hours. Cool, strain, and place in your fridge overnight.
5. Before you are ready to eat, remove the broth from the fridge and skim off any fat

that may have collected. Bring the broth to a simmer and put in the minced ginger.

6. Soak the rice noodles in hot water for ten to twenty minutes or until soft; drain.

7. Blanch the vegetables for approximately one minute. Using a slotted spoon, remove them from the boiling water and shock them in cold water.

8. Flavour the broth to taste with the soy sauce. Flavour the steaks with salt and pepper and grill or broil to your preference.

9. To serve, slice the steaks into fine strips (cutting across the grain) and put them in 6 big bowls. Put in a portion of noodles and vegetables to the bowls and ladle the broth over the top.

Yield: Servings 6

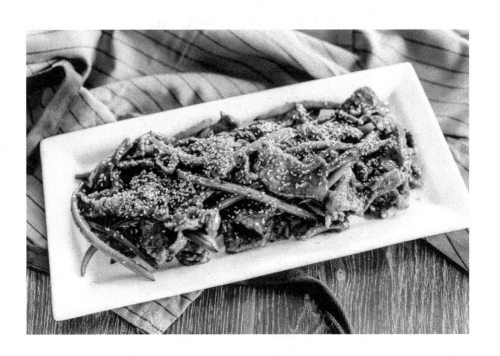

THAI BEEF WITH RICE NOODLES

Ingredients:

- ¼ cup soy sauce
- ½ pound dried rice noodles
- ¾ pound sirloin, trimmed of all fat, washed and patted dry
- 1 pound greens (such as spinach or bok choy), cleaned and slice into ½-inch strips
- 2 eggs, beaten
- 2 tablespoons dark brown sugar
- 2 tablespoons fish sauce
- 2 tablespoons minced garlic
- 5 tablespoons vegetable oil, divided Crushed
- dried red pepper
- flakes to taste Freshly ground
- black pepper Rice
- vinegar to taste

Directions:

1. Cut the meat into two-inch-long, ½–inch-wide strips.
2. Cover the noodles with warm water for five minutes, then drain.
3. In a small container, mix the soy sauce, fish sauce, brown sugar, and black pepper; set aside.
4. Heat a wok or heavy frying pan using high heat. Put in roughly 2 tablespoons of the vegetable oil. Once the oil is hot, but not

smoking, put in the garlic. After stirring for 5 seconds, put in the greens and stir-fry for roughly two minutes; set aside.

5. Put in 2 more tablespoons of oil to the wok. Put in the beef and stir-fry until browned on all sides, approximately 2 minutes; set aside.

6. Heat 1 tablespoon of oil in the wok and put in the noodles. Toss until warmed through, roughly two minutes; set aside.

7. Heat the oil remaining in the wok. Put in the eggs and cook, without stirring until they are set, approximately half a minute. Break up the eggs slightly and mix in the reserved noodles, beef, and greens, and the red pepper flakes. Mix the reserved soy mixture, then put in it to the wok. Toss to coat and heat through. Serve instantly with rice vinegar to drizzle over the top.

Yield: Servings 2–4

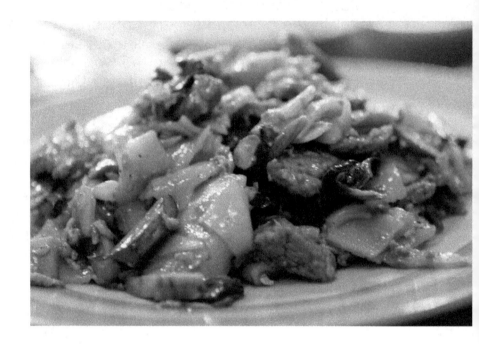

MINTY STIR-FRIED BEEF

Ingredients:

- ¼ cup chopped garlic
- ¼ cup chopped yellow or white onion
- ¼ cup vegetable oil
- ½ cup chopped mint leaves
- ½–¾ cup water
- 1 pound flank steak, cut across the grain into fine strips
- 1 tablespoon sugar
- 3 tablespoons fish sauce
- 7–14 (to taste) serrano chilies, seeded and crudely chopped

Directions:

1. Using a mortar and pestle or a food processor, grind together the chilies, garlic, and onion.
2. Heat the oil on moderate to high heat in a wok or big frying pan. Put in the ground chili mixture to the oil and stir-fry for one to two minutes.
3. Put in the beef and stir-fry until it just starts to brown.
4. Put in the rest of the ingredients, adjusting the amount of water depending on how thick you desire the sauce.
5. Serve with sufficient Jasmine rice.

Yield: Servings 4–6

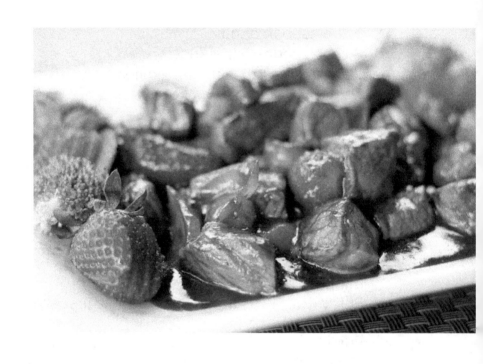

CHILIED BEEF

Ingredients:

- ¼ cup white vinegar
- 1 big red onion, cut
- 1 pound flank steak
- 1 teaspoon dried red pepper flakes
- 2 tablespoons fish sauce
- 3 serrano chilies, stems removed and cut
- 4 scallions, trimmed and thinly cut
- Bibb or romaine lettuce leaves
- Juice of 1 big lime

Directions:

1. Put the cut chilies in a small container with the vinegar; allow it to stand for minimum fifteen minutes.
2. Grill or broil the flank steak to your desired doneness. Remove from the grill, cover using foil, and allow it to stand ten minutes. Thinly slice the streak across the grain.
3. Put the beef slices in a big container. Put in the red onion, scallions, lime juice, and red pepper flakes; toss all of the ingredients together. Cover the dish, place in your fridge, and let marinate for minimum 1 hour.
4. Before you serve, let the beef return to room temperature. Mound the beef on top of lettuce leaves and serve with white rice. Pass the serrano/vinegar sauce separately.

Yield: Servings 4–6

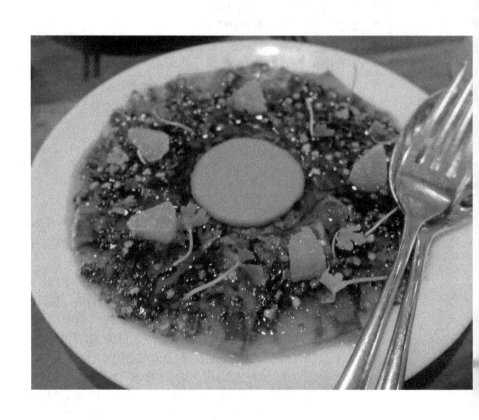

PORK AND EGGPLANT STIR-FRY

Ingredients:

- 3 tablespoons vegetable oil
- ½ pound ground pork
- ½ teaspoon freshly ground pepper
- 1 tablespoon fish sauce
- 1 tablespoon <u>Yellow Bean Sauce</u> <u>(Page 24)</u>
- 1 pound Japanese eggplant, cut into ¼-inch slices ¼ cup
- chicken stock
- 2 tablespoons (or to taste) sugar
- 5–10 cloves garlic, mashed

Directions:

1. Heat the oil in a wok or big frying pan on moderate to high heat. Once the oil is hot, put in the garlic and stir-fry until aromatic, approximately half a minute.
2. Put in the pork and continue to stir-fry until the pork loses its color, approximately one minute.
3. Put in the pepper, fish sauce, bean sauce, and eggplant; cook for a minute.
4. Put in the chicken stock. Continue to stir-fry for a couple of minutes.
5. Mix in the sugar to taste and cook until the eggplant is thoroughly cooked, approximately 2 more minutes.

Yield: Servings 2–4

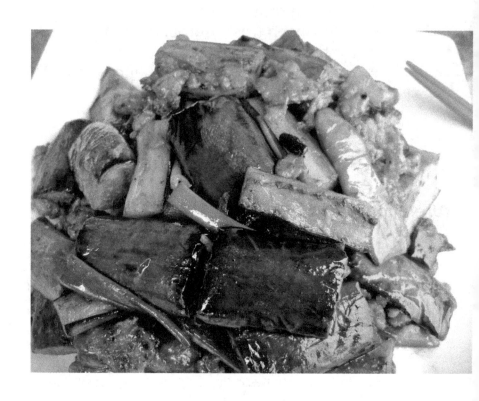

PORK WITH GARLIC AND CRUSHED BLACK PEPPER

Ingredients:

- 4 tablespoons vegetable oil
- 1 pork tenderloin, trimmed of all fat and slice into medallions about ¼-inch thick
- ¼ cup sweet black soy sauce
- 2 tablespoons brown sugar
- 2 tablespoons fish sauce
- 2–2½ teaspoons black peppercorns, crudely ground
- 10–20 garlic cloves, mashed

Directions:

1. Put the garlic and the black pepper in a small food processor and process for a short period of time to make a crude paste; set aside.
2. Heat the oil in a wok or big frying pan on moderate to high heat. Once the oil is hot, put in the garlic-pepper paste and stir-fry until the garlic turns gold.
3. Increase the heat to high and put in the pork medallions; stir-fry for half a minute.
4. Put in the soy sauce and brown sugar, stirring until the sugar is dissolved.
5. Put in the fish sauce and carry on cooking until the pork is thoroughly cooked, approximately another one to two minutes.

Yield: Servings 2

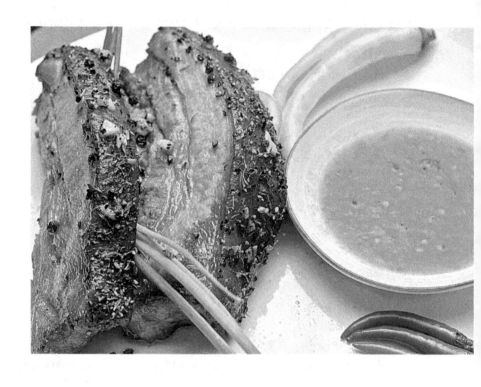

BANGKOK-STYLE ROASTED PORK TENDERLOIN

Ingredients:

- ¼ teaspoon ground cardamom
- ¼ teaspoon ground ginger
- ¼–½ teaspoon freshly ground black pepper
- ½ cup chicken, pork, or vegetable stock, or water
- 1 teaspoon salt
- 2 (1-pound) pork tenderloins,
- trimmed Olive oil

Directions:

1. Put rack on bottom third of the oven, then preheat your oven to 500 degrees.
2. Mix the spices in a small container.
3. Rub each of the tenderloins with half of the spice mixture and a small amount of olive oil. Put the tenderloins in a roasting pan and cook for about ten minutes.
4. Turn the tenderloins over and roast for ten more minutes or until done to your preference.
5. Move the pork to a serving platter, cover using foil, and allow to rest.
6. Pour off any fat that has collected in the roasting pan. Put the pan on the stovetop using high heat and put in the stock (or water). Bring to its boiling point, scraping the bottom of the pan to loosen any

cookedon bits. Sprinkle with salt and pepper to taste.
7. To serve, slice the tenderloins into thin slices. Pour a small amount of the sauce on top, passing more separately at the table.

Yield: Servings 4

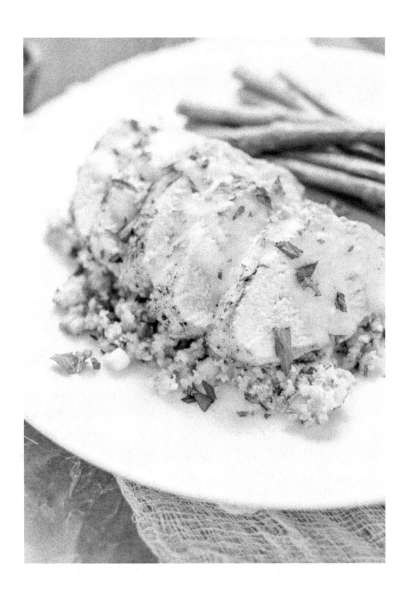

CHIANG MAI BEEF

Ingredients:

- 1 pound lean ground beef
- 1 tablespoon chopped garlic
- 1 tablespoon small dried chilies
- 1 tablespoon vegetable oil
- 2 cups uncooked long-grained rice
- 2 green onions, trimmed and cut
- 3¼ cups water
- 3–4 tablespoons soy sauce
- Fish sauce

Directions:

1. In a big deep cooking pan, bring the water to its boiling point, then mix in the rice. Cover, decrease the heat to low, and cook until the water is absorbed, approximately twenty minutes.
2. Place the cooked rice in a big mixing container and let cool completely.
3. Put in the ground beef and soy sauce to the rice, mixing meticulously. (I find using my hands works best.)
4. Split the rice-beef mixture into 8 to 12 equivalent portions, depending on the size you prefer, and form them into loose balls. Cover each ball in foil, ensuring to secure them well.

5. Steam the rice balls for twenty-five to thirty minutes or until thoroughly cooked.
6. While the rice is steaming, heat the vegetable oil in a small frying pan. Put in the garlic and the dried chilies and sauté until the garlic is golden. Move the garlic and the chilies to a paper towel to drain.
7. To serve, remove the rice packets from the foil, slightly smash them, and put on serving plates. Pass the garlic-chili mixture, the green onions, and the fish sauce separately to be used as condiments at the table.

Yield: Servings 4–6

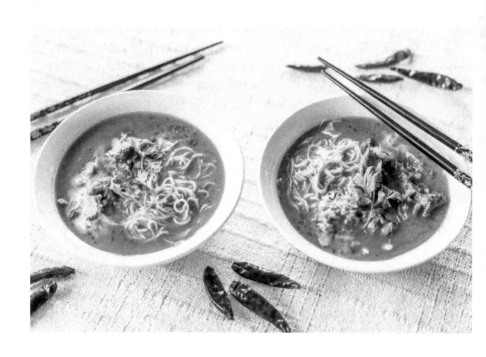

CPSIA information can be obtained
at www.ICGtesting.com
Printed in the USA
BVHW072155270421
605946BV00001BB/179